Weight Training for Golf:

Gain Distance and Improved Accuracy Through Weight Training

By **Carter K Miller**

Copyright

Table of Contents

Introduction to Weight Training for Golf.

Mandy had been playing golf since she was a teen, however she never appeared to be ready to get through to a higher level. She was in every case great, yet all at once never extraordinary. That all changed when she began weight training.Mandy had forever been a fit individual, yet she had never truly given a lot of consideration to her solidarity. She was great at golf, however she generally felt like she was missing something. That is the point at which she chose to begin weight lifting.

From the get go, Mandy had glaring doubts about weight training for golf. She thought it was an exercise in futility. However, as she began to get results, she started to alter her perspective. She was getting more grounded and her golf match-up was improving as well.Mandy was stunned at how her golf swing was changing with the expanded strength and power. She had the option to raise a ruckus around town further and with more exactness. Her scores were improving and she had the option to contend at a higher level.Mandy's weight training routine has turned into a basic piece of her golf match-up. She realizes that she wouldn't be where she is today without it. She is a demonstration of the advantages of weight training and how it can assist you with arriving at your objectives.

weight training for golf is a successful and effective method for further developing your golf match-up. By fortifying your muscles and working on your by and large actual wellness, you can improve as a golf player. weight training is a significant part of a thorough golf work out schedule, and it can assist you with developing fortitude, power, and adaptability. It can likewise assist you with working on your stance, equilibrium, and coordination. weight training can assist with expanding your club head speed, which is significant for creating a more extended, straighter drive. It can likewise assist with working on your general soundness and power during the swing. weight training can likewise assist with decreasing the gamble of injury by expanding your adaptability and equilibrium.

weight training can be custom fitted to explicit region of the body that are significant for golf execution. The center, chest area, and lower body are exceedingly significant for golf and can be focused on with explicit activities. The center muscles help to settle the body during the golf swing and can be prepared with activities like boards and center pivots. The chest area muscles help to create club head speed and can be prepared with activities, for example, chest presses, columns, and horizontal raises. The lower body muscles help to make a strong and stable base for the golf swing and can be prepared with activities like squats, lurches, and step-ups. weight training can be an incredible method for further developing your golf match-up and it ought to be a piece of any thorough golf work out regime. With legitimate preparation and direction, you can turn into a more grounded, all the more impressive golf player.

Benefits of Weight Training for Golf.

Weight training can be a gainful instrument for any golf player as it assists with creating strength, power, and perseverance. weight training can assist with working on a golf player's exhibition by expanding the distance of the golf shot, working on generally soundness and equilibrium, and working on the capacity to produce power during the swing.

Weight training for golf can assist with expanding the general strength of the body, which is significant for the power and speed expected to produce a strong golf swing. By expanding the strength of the muscles in the arms, legs, center, and back, a golf player can produce more power and speed during their swing. This can bring about additional steady shots and longer drives.

As well as speeding up, weight training can likewise assist with expanding security and equilibrium during the golf swing. By fortifying the muscles in the legs, center, and back, a golf player can turn out to be more steady and better adjusted during their swing, which can assist with decreasing the gamble of injury.

In conclusion, weight training can assist with working on a golf player's perseverance. By working on the strength of the muscles in the arms, legs, and center, a golf player can turn out to be better perseverance and have the option to play for longer timeframes without exhaustion setting in. This can assist with working on a golf player's presentation throughout the span of a whole round of golf.

Generally speaking, weight training can be a helpful instrument for any golf player hoping to work on their exhibition. weight training can assist with speeding up, further develop dependability and equilibrium, and further develop perseverance. These elements can assist with working on a golf player's exhibition on the course.

Improved Strength and Power.

Weight training is a compelling method for further developing strength and power. It includes utilizing protection from assemble and reinforce the muscles, which should be possible with loads, machines, or bodyweight works out. When done accurately, weight training can expand strength, power, and bulk.

Strength is the capacity to move a given burden or opposition. Weight training assists with building and fortify the muscles, which can assist you with lifting heavier loads. This expands your solidarity and can assist you with performing better in sports and ordinary exercises.

Power is the capacity to rapidly apply force. weight training assists with creating unstable power by speeding up at which muscles can produce force. This can assist you with working

on your presentation in sports, as well as exercises like
running, bouncing, and tossing.

Weight training additionally assists with expanding bulk.
Muscles give the body serious areas of strength for an and
support for different exercises, like running and hopping.
Having more bulk can assist you with performing better in
everyday exercises, as well as sports.

In general, weight training is a viable method for further
developing strength, power, and bulk. It can assist you with
performing better in sports and ordinary exercises, and will
assist you with remaining solid and fit.

Improved Flexibility and Mobility

weight training is a very compelling method for further
developing adaptability and portability. Power lifting, when
done accurately and securely, puts strain on the body's
muscles and joints and assists with extending them. The
strain assists with extending the muscles, which then, at that
point, expands the joints' scope of movement and adaptability.
weight training can likewise assist with further developing
muscle coordination, which can assist with further developing
stance and equilibrium.

weight training can likewise assist with further developing
scope of movement and portability. This is on the grounds that
when a muscle is prepared, it becomes more grounded and
more steady, and this solidness can assist with working on the

scope of movement of the joints. The expanded muscle strength can likewise assist with supporting the joints and make them more steady, which can assist with further developing portability.

weight training is an incredible method for further developing adaptability and versatility, as it can assist with extending the muscles and increment their scope of movement. It can likewise assist with further developing muscle coordination, solidness, and stance, which can assist with further developing portability.

Improved Balance and Stability.

weight training for golf can further develop equilibrium and steadiness by reinforcing the muscles and joints utilized in the golf swing. By performing activities like squats, deadlifts, and jumps, the muscles in the legs, hips, and center become more grounded and better ready to balance out the body during the swing. Strength preparing likewise assists with expanding balance by working on the coordination between the various muscles utilized in the golf swing. Moreover, customary weight training reinforces the postural muscles, which can assist with diminishing the gamble of injury and further develop pose. At long last, weight training for golf can likewise assist with expanding adaptability, which can assist with further developing equilibrium and dependability during the golf swing. In general, weight training for golf can essentially

further develop equilibrium and strength during the golf swing,
making it one of the main parts of any golf player's
preparation program.

Types of Weight Training for Golf.

1. Core Strength Training – Core strength training isintended to work on a golf player's capacity to produce power by fortifying the muscles of the storage compartment. Activities like boards, crunches, and back augmentations can be utilized to reinforce the center muscles, which will assist the golf player with producing power from their middle.

2. Plyometric Training – Plyometric training is designed to increase explosive power. Explosive power is important in golf because it's needed for a powerful swing. Exercises such as medicine ball throws, jump squats, and box jumps can be used to increase explosive power.

3. Upper Body Strength Training – Upper body strength training is designed to strengthen the muscles of the upper body. To strengthen the upper body, exercises like lat pull-downs, shoulder presses, and bicep curls can be done. The golfer will be able to generate more club head speed and distance thanks to this.

4. Lower Body Strength Training – Lower body strength training is intended to expand the strength of the lower body muscles. Activities like squats, lurches, and leg expansions can be utilized to increment lower body strength. This will assist the golf player with creating more power and steadiness during their golf swing.

5. Speed and Agility training - Speed and spryness preparing is intended to build a golf player's dexterity and speed. Activities, for example, stepping stool drills, cone penetrates, and runs can be utilized to speed up and deftness. This will assist the golf player with creating more club head speed and exactness.

 6. Resistance training - Opposition preparing is intended to expand a golf player's solidarity, power, and perseverance. Activities, for example, opposition band works out, hand weight works out, and bodyweight activities can be utilized to increment obstruction. This will assist the golf player with producing more power and perseverance all through their whole swing.

Developing a Weight Training Program for Golf

The following steps will help you develop an effective weight training program tailored to your individual needs and help you achieve your fitness goals.

1. Distinguish your objectives: Would you say you are hoping to increment strength, assemble muscle, or work on your general wellness? Understanding what you desire to accomplish with weight training will assist you with making a program custom fitted to your singular requirements.

2. Pick the right activities: Select activities that focus on the muscles you need to deal with and utilize legitimate structure while lifting. Work on compound developments like squats, presses, and deadlifts to accomplish the best outcomes.

3. Set up a timetable: Lay out a predictable gym routine everyday practice and choose how long each week you'll give to power lifting. Make a point to permit sufficient rest days between exercises so your body can recuperate.

4. Put forth reasonable objectives: Put forth practical objectives and consider your ongoing wellness level and experience. Intend to expand how much weight you're lifting over the long run and endeavor to meet your objectives.

5. Screen progress: Keep tabs on your development by keeping a preparation log and measure your advancement concerning weight, reps, and length. This will assist you with understanding how your body is answering the program and change it depending on the situation.

6. Adapt: As you progress, make acclimations to your program. Increment the weight, reps, or sets depending on the situation and make it a point to change around your daily schedule or add new activities to keep it fascinating.

7. Remain inspired: Track down ways of remaining propelled and stay reliable with your program. Pay attention to music, read rousing books, or get an exercise mate to assist you with keeping focused.

8. Center around Center Strength: One of the main components of an effective weight training program for golf is center strength. The center muscles are answerable for creating power, keeping up with balance, and controlling your swing. Center around practices that focus on the center, like boards, crunches, and rotational developments.

9. Consolidate Plyometrics: Plyometric activities can assist with expanding power and dangerousness in the golf swing. Center around works out, for example, hopping squats and box bounces, that require speedy, strong developments.

10. Consolidate Versatility Work: Portability is a frequently ignored part of golf execution, yet it is fundamental for forestalling injury and keeping up with great structure. Invest energy performing portability drills to expand scope of movement and adaptability.

11. Recuperation: Remember to give your body time to recuperate after every exercise. Rest and recuperation are fundamental to forestall injury and permit the body to adjust and get to the next level.

By following these tips, you can create an effective weight training program for golf. Remember to take time to assess your goals, choose a program that is appropriate for you, and focus on core strength and mobility. With consistent effort and dedication, you can improve your golf game and take your performance to the next level.

Proper form and Techniques for weight training exercises

1. Squats: Begin by remaining with feet marginally more extensive than shoulder width separated. Twist at the knees and hips, then lower yourself into a squat position. Ensure that your knees stay despite your toes and that your good faith is kept straight all through the movement. When you arrive at the lower part of the squat, press through your heels to get back to the beginning position. Perform 3 arrangements of 8-12 redundancies.

2. Thrusts: Start by remaining with feet hip-width separated. Step forward with one leg, twisting the two knees to 90 degrees. Ensure that your front knee stays despite your toes and that your good faith knee remains nearby the ground. Push through your front heel to get back to the beginning position. Perform 3 arrangements of 8-12 reiterations on every leg.

3. Step-Ups: Begin by remaining before a stage or seat. Move forward onto the step with one leg, making a point to keep your back straight all through the movement. Press through your heel to get back to the beginning position. Perform 3 arrangements of 8-12 redundancies on every leg.

4. Medication Ball Revolutions: Start by remaining with feet marginally more extensive than shoulder-width separated. Hold a medication ball before your chest. Turn your middle aside and afterward back to the middle. Perform 3 arrangements of 8-12 redundancies on each side.

5. Chest Press: Lie on a level seat with your feet level on the floor. Hold a couple of free weights at shoulder-width separated. Press the loads straight up, then, at that point, lower them back to the beginning position. Ensure that your elbows remain nearby your sides all through the movement. Perform 3 arrangements of 8-12 reiterations.

6. Lat Pulldowns: Connect a bar to a link machine. Plunk down on the seat and handle the bar at shoulder-width separated. Pull the bar down to your chest, then return to the beginning position. Make a point to keep your elbows near your sides all through the movement. Perform 3 arrangements of 8-12 redundancies.

Weight Training Safety.

Weight training can be a great way to stay healthy, but it is important to take safety precautions when lifting weights.
First, make sure to always use proper form. It is better to lift lighter weights with correct form than heavier weights with incorrect form. If you are unsure of how to do an exercise correctly, ask a trainer or do some research online.
Second, always warm up before lifting. This will help prevent injury and prepare your body for the workout.
Third, use a spotter when lifting heavy weights. This will ensure you don't injure yourself if you are unable to complete a rep.
Fourth, take breaks when needed. Don't push yourself too hard, and if you feel any pain, stop and rest.
Finally, make sure you are using the correct equipment. Use the appropriate weight for your level of strength and make sure the equipment is in good condition.

By following these tips, you can stay safe and enjoy the benefits of weight training.

Exercises and Stretches that Help in Increasing Flexibility and Range of Motion

1. Standing Ride Stretch: Stand with your feet more extensive than shoulder-width separated and toes marginally called attention to. Gradually lower your chest towards your toes and hold for 30 seconds.

2. Standing Quad Stretch: Remaining on one leg, hold the lower leg of the other leg behind you and pull it towards your butt cheek. Hold for 30 seconds and switch legs.

3. Situated Hamstring Stretch: Sit on the ground with the two legs reached out before you. Reach forward and hold your toes for 30 seconds.

4. Standing Toe Contact: Stand with your feet shoulder-width separated. Twist forward at the hips, keeping your knees marginally bowed, and reach towards your toes. Hold for 30 seconds.

5. Rushes: Step in the right direction with one foot and lower your body until your front knee is bowed at a 90-degree point. Hold for 30 seconds. Switch legs.

6. Hip Flexor Stretch: Stoop on the ground and present one knee with the goal that it is bowed at a 90-degree point. Push your hips forward and hold for 30 seconds. Switch legs.

7. Stomach Crunches: Lie on your back with your knees bowed and your feet level on the ground. Twist your shoulders off the ground and hold for 3-5 seconds. Lower and rehash.

8. Wall Chest Stretch: Stand confronting a wall and put your hands on it at shoulder-level. Gradually incline forward, extending your chest muscles. Hold for 30 seconds.

Benefits of proper nutrition and hydration for golf performance.

For golf performance, proper nutrition and hydration are essential. Golfers can boost their energy, concentration, and physical and mental endurance by eating the right foods and drinking enough fluids.

When it comes to the mental and physical aspects of golf performance, nutrition plays a crucial role. You can get the energy, nutrients, and vitamins you need to perform at your best when you eat a well-balanced diet rich in proteins, carbohydrates, and fats. During a round of golf, eating foods with a low glycemic index can help provide sustained energy. Consuming foods high in antioxidants, like fruits and vegetables, can aid in recovery and reduce oxidative stress.

Golf performance is also impacted by hydration. Drinking an adequate number of liquids assists with keeping up with the body's liquid equilibrium and forestalls lack of hydration. Fatigue, muscle weakness, and decreased mental focus are all symptoms of dehydration. Remaining hydrated keeps up with smartness and actual endurance for further developed execution.

Golfers may also benefit from maintaining and achieving a healthy body weight by drinking enough fluids and eating the right foods. Diets high in fiber and low in saturated fat, cholesterol, and sodium aid in weight loss and lower the risk of chronic disease. Playing golf can also be made safer by eating a healthy diet and staying at a healthy weight.

In synopsis, legitimate sustenance and hydration are fundamental for golf execution. The energy, nutrients, and vitamins needed to perform at their best can be obtained by eating a diet that is well-balanced and contains the appropriate amounts of proteins, carbohydrates, and fats. For improved physical and mental endurance, drinking enough fluids helps to maintain the body's fluid balance and prevent dehydration. Having a healthy diet and staying in good shape can help you play golf without getting hurt.

conclusion

 Weight training is an essential component of golf fitness. It can help you improve your game by increasing power, strength, flexibility, and range of motion. Additionally, it may assist in lowering the likelihood of golf-related injuries, such as lower back pain. Weight training can also help you swing better and be more accurate by improving your balance, coordination, and stability.

Each golfer's needs should be taken into consideration when devising weight training routines. It's important to choose exercises that target the muscles used in the golf swing because different exercises work different muscle groups. Flexibility and mobility drills should come before strength training to warm up the muscles and increase range of motion. For most exercises, reps should be between 8 and 12, with power-based exercises using heavier weights for lower reps.

To avoid injury while performing weight training exercises, proper form is essential. During the exercise, it's also important to breathe deeply and maintain good posture. Additionally, it is essential to strike a good balance between endurance and strength training.

Last but not least, it is essential to comprehend the significance of recovery. For the muscles to recover and grow, they need adequate rest and nutrition. You'll be able to fuel your workouts and have the energy you need to perform at your best if you eat a well-balanced diet that includes enough protein and carbohydrates.

In conclusion, a golf fitness program may include weight training as an efficient and beneficial component. It can help you improve your game by increasing power, strength, flexibility, range of motion, and balance. However, in order to get the most out of weight training, proper form, maintaining good posture and breathing, and getting enough rest and food are essential. When done correctly, weight training can help you improve your golf game and lower your risk of injury.